YOUR KNOWLEDGE HAS VALUE

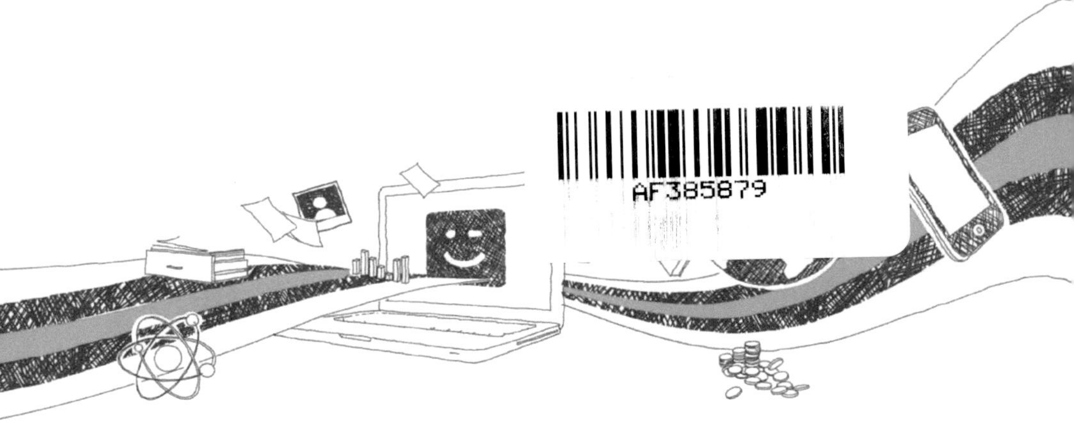

- We will publish your bachelor's and
  master's thesis, essays and papers

- Your own eBook and book -
  sold worldwide in all relevant shops

- Earn money with each sale

Upload your text at www.GRIN.com
and publish for free

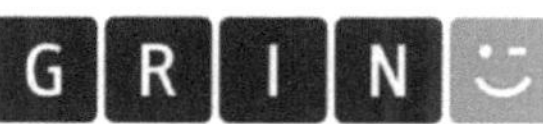

Nassef Adiong

The Dynamics, Magnitude and Scope of MRSA Health Care Associated Infection Concomitant with the Politics in the NHS on the Health Act 2006

From Varied Theories, Policy to Recommended Practices

GRIN Publishing

Bibliographic information published by the German National Library:

The German National Library lists this publication in the National Bibliography; detailed bibliographic data are available on the Internet at http://dnb.dnb.de .

Imprint:

Copyright © 2008 GRIN Verlag, Open Publishing GmbH
Print and binding: Books on Demand GmbH, Norderstedt Germany
ISBN: 978-3-640-73675-1

This book at GRIN:

http://www.grin.com/en/e-book/160433/the-dynamics-magnitude-and-scope-of-mrsa-health-care-associated-infection

The Dynamics, Magnitude and Scope of MRSA Health Care Associated Infection Concomitant with the Politics in the NHS on the Health Act 2006: From Varied Theories, Policy to Recommended Practices

Nassef M. Adiong

In the indicated foreword letter of Janice Stevens (2008), she announced the target of the Department of Health to halve the number of Methicillin-resistant Staphylococcus aureus (MRSA) bacteraemia by this year. As an infection control nurse, this monograph will discuss about MRSA which requires a stringent study to mitigate and control such perpetrated example of a Healthcare Acquired Infections (HCAI) in cognizant with the implemented Health Act 2006 of the National Health Service (NHS) and in relation to the underlying theories and practices in explaining the policy and how will this affects the MRSA issue-area with the help of digesting NHS geopolitics.

Epidemiological issue of interest contextualized with past, current and future saliency: Understanding the dynamics of MRSA, its nature to diagnostic treatment and preventions (First Section)

MRSA was discovered in 1961 in the United Kingdom (UK) that is alternately known in the public as a "superbug" in the wikipedia's page (2008), while the MRSA Action UK (2008) opined that this is a strain that is very similar to any other strain of Staphylococcus aureus. That is, some healthy people are carriers, and some develop the types of infections. The observed increased mortality in countries like United States and UK was among MRSA-infected patients that resulted to the increased underlying morbidity. According to www.nhs.uk page (2008), MRSA infections are more difficult to treat due to adamant antibiotic resistance of the bacteria. A prevalent cause is when an MRSA bacteria spread from person-to-person contact with someone positive with MRSA infection, or who was colonized by the bacteria.

MRSA infections are most common in Hospital staff and members. The reason for this premise is that they often have an entry point for bacteria to get into their body, such as a surgical wound, a catheter, or an intravenous tube. However, MRSA is treatable which will depend on the bacterium you're infected with – Staphylococcus aureus (SA) or only colonized. This treatment is in the form of given antibiotics, which you have to complete the course. According to Hawkes (2007) that a quick test for the drug-resistant bacterium MRSA has helped a London hospital to cut infection rates 40 percent in a single year. In addition, the test was able to detect MRSA in nasal swabs in two hours with the help of effective new technologies, such as rapid tests which can help speed the selection of appropriate interventions. Additionally in Verar's thesis (2008), MRSA has been a significant nosocomical pathogen globally due to its ability to efficiently resist lactam antibiotics and a high expression of heterogeneity among MRSA suggests that confirmatory test by screening is essential for verification.

This is in line with the study done by Keshtgar et al (2007) that aims to establish a feasible and cost-effectiveness report on rapid molecular screening for hospital that have had acquired MRSA in surgical patients. Consequently, the study showed that MRSA positive patients will undergo a suppression therapy of mupirocin nasal ointment and undiluted chlorhexidine gluconate bodywash that resulted into a significant reduction in staphylococcal bacteraemia during the screening period, although a causal link cannot be established is the caveat of the research work. Similarly, a program perpetuated by Dr. Rao (2008) requiring all emergency admissions in University Hospital Lewisham, which has proven to be highly effective strategy for detection of MRSA colonization, has enabled the trust to identify the origin of MRSA-colonized patients, and has informed their strategy to manage high-risk groups appropriately.

A relative study did by Klevens (2007) uses a surveillance methodology in the presence of Active Bacterial Core system (ABCs) that detected incidence rates and estimated number of invasive MRSA infections and in-hospital deaths among patients. In return, the study concludes that invasive MRSA infection affects certain populations disproportionately. On the other hand, Stevens (2008) stipulates that the Department of Health have issued mandatory HCAI surveillance system in the form of Clostridium difficile and have implemented different capacities i.e. changing practice in a sustainable way which requires learning specifically from the causes of infection. The root cause analysis tool was designed by the National Patient Safety Agency (NPSA) to enable teams to learn how infections were caused and how to plan so that they do not re-occur.

In McCaughey's book (2006), a staunch anti-infection death advocate of the Committee to Reduce Infection Deaths, have established new skeletal recommendations under the Specialist Advisory Committee on Antimicrobial Resistance (established to advise the government):

- Screen all patients admitted to "high risk" units, such as the ICU, cardiothoracic, orthopedic, and burn units.
- Minimize movements of MRSA positive patients.
- Use gowns and disposable aprons when treating MRSA positive patients.]
- Launder privacy curtains or use disposable curtains.
- Decontaminate trolleys and wheelchairs after patient use.
- Before surgery, attempt to decolonize MRSA positive patients.
- In the recovery area, segregate MRSA positive patients.

This was deliberately discussed by Siegel (2006), a total concise control interventions were introduced in explaining and further elaborating the above skeletal recommendations. These included administrative support, judicious use of antimicrobials, surveillance (routine and enhanced), Standard and Contact Precautions, environmental measures, education and decolonization. These interventions were applied in various combinations and degrees of intensity, with differences in outcome. These intervening recommendations were grouped into seven (7) categories, as studies shown by Siegel:

1. Administrative support. Interventions that require administrative support include:

a) Implementing system changes to ensure prompt and effective communications e.g., computer alerts to identify patients previously known to be colonized/infected with MRSA;

b) Providing the necessary number and appropriate placement of hand washing sinks and alcohol-containing hand rub dispensers in the facility;

c) Maintaining staffing levels appropriate to the intensity of care required; and

d) Enforcing adherence to recommended infection control practices (e.g., hand hygiene, Standard and Contact Precautions) for MRSA control.

2. Education. The focus of this intervention was to encourage a behavioral change through improved understanding of the problem MRSA that the facility was trying to control. Whether the desired change involved hand hygiene, antimicrobial prescribing patterns, or other outcomes, enhancing understanding and creating a culture that supported and promoted the desired behavior, were viewed as essential to the success of the intervention.

3. Judicious use of antimicrobial agents. While a comprehensive review of antimicrobial stewardship is beyond the scope of this guideline, recommendations for control of MRSA must include attention to judicious antimicrobial use. Limiting antimicrobial use alone may fail to control resistance due to a combination of factors; including

    a) the relative effect of antimicrobials on providing initial selective pressure, compared to perpetuating resistance once it has emerged;

    b) inadequate limits on usage; or

    c) insufficient time to observe the impact of this intervention.

Strategies for influencing antimicrobial prescribing patterns within healthcare facilities include education; formulary restriction; prior-approval programs, including pre-approved indications; automatic stop orders; academic interventions to counteract pharmaceutical influences on prescribing patterns; antimicrobial cycling; computer-assisted management programs; and active efforts to remove redundant antimicrobial combinations.

4. MRSA surveillance. Surveillance is a critically important component of any MRSA control program, allowing detection of newly emerging pathogens, monitoring epidemiologic trends, and measuring the effectiveness of interventions. Multiple MRSA surveillance strategies have been employed, ranging from surveillance of clinical microbiology laboratory results obtained as part of routine clinical care, to detect asymptomatic colonization. The following were the different surveillance strategies:

    a) Antibiograms

    b) MRSA Incidence Based on Clinical Culture Results

    c) Molecular typing of MRSA isolates

    d) Surveillance for MRSA by Detecting Asymptomatic Colonization

5. Infection Control Precautions. Standard Precautions have an essential role in preventing MRSA transmission, even in facilities that use Contact Precautions for patients with an identified MRSA. Colonization with MRSA is frequently undetected; even surveillance cultures may fail to identify colonized persons due to lack of sensitivity, laboratory deficiencies, or intermittent colonization due to antimicrobial therapy. Therefore, Standard Precautions must be used in order to prevent transmission from potentially colonized patients. Hand hygiene is an important component of Standard Precautions.

On the other hand, the Contact Precautions are intended to prevent transmission of infectious agents, including epidemiologically important microorganisms, which are transmitted by direct or indirect contact with the patient or the patient's environment. A single-patient room is preferred for patients who require Contact Precautions. When a single-patient room is not available, consultation with infection control is necessary to assess the various risks associated with other patient placement options (e.g. chortling or keeping the patient with an existing roommate).

6. Environmental measures. The potential role of environmental reservoirs, such as surfaces and medical equipment, in the transmission of MRSA has been the subject of several reports. While environmental cultures are not routinely recommended, environmental cultures were used in several studies to document contamination, and led to interventions that included the use of dedicated non-critical medical equipment, assignment of dedicated cleaning personnel to the affected patient care unit, and increased cleaning and disinfection of frequently-touched surfaces (e.g., bedrails, charts, bedside commodes, doorknobs).

7. Decolonization. This entails treatment of persons colonized with MRSA, to eradicate carriage of that organism through several regimens that include topical mupirocin alone or in combination with orally administered antibiotics (e.g., rifampin in combination with trimethoprim-sulfamethoxazole or ciprofloxacin) plus the use of an antimicrobial soap for bathing. Decolonization regimens are not sufficiently effective to warrant routine use. Therefore, most healthcare facilities have limited the use of decolonization to MRSA outbreaks, or other high prevalence situations, especially those affecting special-care units. Several factors limit the utility of this control measure on a widespread basis:

1) Identification of candidates for decolonization requires surveillance cultures;

2) Candidates receiving decolonization treatment must receive follow-up cultures to ensure eradication; and

3) Decolonization with the same strain, initial colonization with a mupirocin-resistant strain, and emergence of resistance to mupirocin during treatment can occur.

The NHS politics on The Health Act 2006: Outlining the preordained principles and conceptualizations of the embedded varied theories (Second Section)

In Milio (1991), health policy sees human health in an ecological relationship with all else in our natural and human-made habitats. It is relevant to both high- and low-income countries although its priorities will defer in different nations. Simply put Health public policy that sets the range of possibilities for the choices made by public and private organizations. From the attached brief on Options Paper on Establishing a Decolonization Service for Pre-elective Surgical Patients Screened as MRSA Positive, it was conceived that in 2006 the Department of Health published the "Health Act; the Code of Practice for the Prevention and Control of Health Care Associated Infections." Its aim is to help NHS bodies plan and implement how they can prevent and control HCAI. In addition, "Saving Lives, reducing infection and implementing clean and safe care," provides the tools and resources for Trusts to do this, including the Essential Steps framework for Primary Care Trusts (PCTs).

Organizations must ensure they comply with the Code of Practice and implement best practice from Saving Lives. The 2008-09 NHS Operating Framework states that although no healthcare system can be entirely risk free we must do more to reduce the rate of HCAIs and that organizations need to take particular action in 2008/09. Trusts must ensure progress in relation to reducing MRSA through maintaining the annual number of MRSA bloodstream infections at less than half the number in 2003/04. It also states that Trusts must also achieve the 18 week access target for elective surgery as one of the top five national priorities.

The current understanding is that patients requiring decolonization will not be suspended on the surgical waiting list whilst decolonization is carried out.

All of these were realized from the establishment and implementation of The Health Act 2006. Which according to Nicholson (2007), its postulated premise is undertaken in the principle of "The prevention and control of HCAI as a priority for all parts of the NHS" As a result it is essential that all hospital staff are aware of the correct procedures or policies to reduce the onward transmission of MRSA. Good hygiene (Standard Infection Control Precautions) particularly in the form of simple every day precautions, is all that is required to prevent the spread of MRSA. Thorough hand decontamination between caring for people, and whenever necessary (before and after all patient contacts), has been shown to be the single most important measure in reducing cross infection. As Nicholson further stipulates, this policy applies to all staff working in any PCTs units involved with patient services in either the healthcare setting or patients own homes, including bank, agency, students and volunteers. Individuals have the responsibility to comply with this policy and report any incidents/risks that occur. PCTs Managers have the responsibility to ensure personnel comply with this policy and for ensuring adequate hand hygiene resources are available at all times.

In Harrison et al (1990), revisiting theories under the ambit of health policy, ***Neo-Elite theory*** is often concerned with occupational elites through the personage of group of doctors, hospital consultants, in obstructing the implementation of national priorities in health care and resource allocation, in evading managerial control, and in avoiding a potentially threatening debate about the evaluation of services. While on ***Neo-Marxist theory*** the elites are constructed to the class structure of the capitalist state. The interest is not merely scholastic concern with the categorization of particular occupations into social classes but rather an attempt to investigate the functions of elites in supporting or challenging the capitalist state. In this theory, it has been believed that there would be an eventual 'crisis of the welfare state'; at some risk oversimplification, the argument runs as follows. Demand for welfare state expenditure rises over time, as a result of a number of factors; demographic changes and public expectations are amongst those frequently cited. The government cannot easily respond to these concerns however, since to cut welfare state expenditure world risk offending public opinion, that is, threatens its legitimate function.

In reference to neo-Marxist theory, I would like to emphasized the general practitioner (GP) fundholders negotiating contracts with the PCT that provide services, which has elected to hold its own funds for negotiating contracts and purchasing a range of health care services for its patients reflecting in the criterion laid by the ICN, which is heavily involved in monitoring quality and performance of the acute trust and care delivered in primary care. Baines and Whynes (1996) uses to analyze the differences in characteristics between existing fundholding, non-fundholding practices, and negotiated contracts delivered for the PCT services. Contracts revealed to be more likely negotiated in the presence of both parties than non-fundholders, which may meet a number of the various quality criteria embodied by central government following the 1990 NHS Act, for example, with respect to the dilemmas of prescribing cost control, minor surgery, cervical screening uptake, and HCAI mitigational processes. Thus, it employed to forecast that the contracts lead to poor predictions as it suggests the existence of a structural break in the characteristics of both parties (GP fundholders and the PCT) other than non-fundholders. It represents a support to the existence of selection bias in fundholding, although further logistic negotiation reveals a form of such bias.

Kay A. (2002) presented that the GP fundholding scheme was introduced as part of the Conservative government's 1991 NHS reforms and abolished by the Thatcher's Labor government that may have had stimulated competition between the providers in the "internal market.". They contend that the scheme was introduced and abolished without policy-makers having any valid evidence of its effects. In particular, it focuses on the salient features of the decision to abolish. These were: (a) that it was not based on evidence; (b) that it came relatively soon after the introduction of the scheme; and (c) the GP fundholding scheme was voluntary and increasing numbers of GPs were being recruited. The overtly political nature of the introduction of GP fundholding is already well documented and is important in understanding the lack of evidence involved in the development of the fundholding scheme.

This was posited on the 'Plan for Social Security' of the Beveridge Report particularly in the expenditure's scheme. The actual incomes and by consequence the normal standards of expenditure of different sections of the population differ greatly for higher standards, which is primarily the function of the individual that is to say, it is a matter for free choice and voluntary insurance. But the State should make sure that its measures leave room and encouragement. The financial burden of HCAI's 'The National Audit Office' reported an estimate of over a billion a year. The successful increasing litigation for MRSA acquired infections and the DH knee jerk response to screen all elective surgery by 31st March and all other surgery by 2011. These may imply on the health policy in the following assertions:

- Comprehensive health and rehabilitation services for prevention and cure of disease and restoration of capacity for work, available to all members of the community;
- Social insurance and national assistance organized by the State.
- Incapacity for household duties, met by provision of paid help in illness as part of treatment.

Furthermore, from the attached data of executive summary and key benefits in the business case template of decolonization of MRSA plus elective patients, an outline was made detailing the financial, clinical, and organizational key risks:

- This is a "must do" from the priorities laid out in the 2008-09 NHS Operating Framework- the PCT cannot afford to ignore establishing a suitable service.
- Patients will experience a delay in 18 week access to necessary surgical treatment.
- The numbers of potential MRSA positive patients is an estimate so the actual numbers may be higher or lower than this impacting on the overall financial costs and potential efficiency of the service we establish.
- The potential demands and costs to MCH in option 3 are difficult to quantify.
- There will be increased morbidity and mortality associated with MRSA bacteraemia for patients identified as MRSA positive, but not decolonized promptly once suspended from the elective waiting list.

The affordability and costs were also outlined from the template. Based on the estimated numbers of MRSA positive patients in 2008-09 (4640) the basic costs of decolonization- prescribing and re-screening- are:

- Decolonization per patient: £42.57
- Total decolonization costs: £197,524 (42.57x4640)
- Re-screening per patient: £36 (£12/screenx3)
- Total re-screening costs: £167,040 (36x4640)

My prism here, is that even within the scope of theories describing proportionate appropriations on Health Act 2006, it does not explain everything. Some important changes, such as the introduction of general management, sprang from the actions of the individuals and to this extent are quite uncomprehending in terms of any of the theoretical approaches This does not mean, however, that such changes might not be the appropriate subject of some other theory, which would be less general, but might relate to it in the same kind of hierarchical fashion. Consequently, Allsop (1995) described politics in NHS as extraneously exasperating between in two powerful interest groups, the government and the medical profession. Indeed, it has been argued that UK health politics is corporatist in style. This is interpreted in a thesis, a process of what they call 'mutual partisan adjustment', occurs. In other words, the various structured-interest groups adjust to each other in shaping policy within a framework of accepted conventions.

The corporatist approach according to Allsop, tends to take an over-simple view of health care politics with little recognition that the political interplay of groups may vary. Shifts in health care policy and the mode of delivery is not a single explanation for policy change, rather a number of factors contribute but appear in different combinations. The ideology and political values of the government; the state of the economy; demographic change; the possibilities offered by technology as well as more apocalyptic factors such as war, scandals and epidemics have all been shown to play a part in policy modification. Subsequent example i.e. Conservative Party monetarists clearly saw excessive public expenditures as lying at the heart of economic difficulties in the UK. It was argued that economic growth rates must be improved before welfare services could likewise be upgraded. Thus the attainment of economic goals as given priority over social policy goals. This was the view that underpinned the policy shifts of the last decade.

This proposition was questioned by Folland et al (2001), that health economics in health care is paramount that attaining economic and social goals. They said that the study of health economics proves important and interesting in three interrelated ways: (1) the size of the contribution of the health sector to the overall economy, (2) the national policy concerns resulting from the importance many people attach to the economic problems they face in pursuing and maintaining their health, and (3) the fact that many other health issues have a substantial economic element. They even suggest that health care has many distinctive features, but that is not unique in any of them. What is unique perhaps is the combination of features and even the sheer number of them. These are the characterizations or features in health care: the presence and extent of uncertainty on the demand side and the supply side, the prominence of insurance, the problems of information, the large role of nonprofit firms, the restrictions on competition, the role of equity and need, and the government subsidies and public provision. Can we apply these features on the politics in NHS?

Harrison et al (1992) will answer the posited query; it is a matter of key concepts in the politics of NHS, relating to the concept of power as exercised when, as means of influence, the threat of a sanction is made, thus this sanction can, of course, be the withholding of a reward which would otherwise have been given. The logical corollary of power is, therefore, freedom from dependence or autonomy. A power relationship exists when: (a) there is a conflict over values or course of action between A and B; (b) B comply with A's wishes; and (c) B does so because he is fearful that A will deprive him of a value(s) which he regards more highly than those which would have been achieved by noncompliance. However, politics is not all about conflict and power. Puzzlement and uncertainty according to Harrison are common features in respect of policy-making and implementation. The contribution of the 'health problem' to puzzlement stems from a series of fundamental uncertainties. The health status of a population as well as the means of improving it remains cloudy. The author even included a concept on Post-Fordist Model, which describes NHS politics as hybrid of task and role with elements of person culture typically networking in a contractual relationship within the broad framework of a strategic plan.

Evaluating the politics in NHS performances consonance with the Health Act 2006 through the mitigational strategies of MRSA mentioned in the first section: Noting probable recommendations on NHS based on theoretical approaches determined in the second section? (Third Section)

To implement total quality management of the policy on Health Act 2006 for the controlling and mitigating MRSA infections, there must be a firm commitment from the leadership of the NHS to change their former way of doing business. The role of the leader is valuable. Leaders must continually ask: Do our quality systems support continuous improvement and innovation? If not, what changes must be made? How can we better align our organization to meet the needs of our community particularly in the health sector? The concept of Hospital workforce empowerment and involvement is also critical. Customer-focused organizations understand the requirements of both internal and external customers.

Hence, according to Gaucher and Coffey (1993), there are several key implementation factors such as:

- *Creation of a Common Direction.* The goal is to align the NHS behind the mission, vision, and goals. This allows each person to understand how his or her job contributes to organizational success. Alignment creates organizational synergy.
- *Cultural Change.* The leaders within NHS must personally model the new behaviors, or the transformation will lack energy and credibility.
- *Communication.* The first step to improvement is flowcharting of all critical processes so that an effective communication will be essential to the success of the quality initiative.
- *Integration.* Requires the integration of a customer-focused continuous improvement philosophy, analytical knowledge and skills, and interpersonal knowledge and skills.
- *Achieving a Balanced Approach.* There must be a balance of analytical, humanistic, and customer-oriented skills.
- *The Role of Innovation and Creativity.* There should be creativity training for those who would like to develop a dual focus on improvement and innovation.

In the Health Act 2006, four scenarios were discussed for health care by Morrison (2000): (1) *Community Care,* wherein local and state governments are willing partners in community-based reform; (2) *Medicare Choice for All,* low interest rates, the movement of baby boomers from being net debtors to net savers, and continued competitive pressure to raise productivity through technological and organizational innovation combine to fuel an investment boom; (3) *Ugly Recession,* this is a selfish health care system; those who are doing OK don't complain. But on one in their right mind would say that it's the best way for a nation i.e. politicians won't touch it, NHS doesn't care about it anymore, and those in the game squabble over what there is. (4) *Adam Smith Beats Karl Marx – Health Care as Financial Services,* for health care the lessons from financial services are taken to heart by employers, the managed care industry, providers, and consumers alike. As Morrison would put it, there are seven key changes take place:

1) *The shift from defined benefit to contribution is complete.* For a typical employee, health benefits come in a form of monthly allowance to be applied to any number of health and wealth options as well as plans that have restricted health coverage but expanded long term care and disability coverage.

2) *There is regulatory support for new products.* Pushes for regulatory changes that make health care operate more like other financial services, such as mutual funds and mortgages.

3) *The health care value chain becomes like that of financial services.* In the new world, the people who sell you the loan on its balance sheet, bundle up like loans into standardized blocks that they resell to another party; meanwhile the processing and administration of the loan payments are done by a third party.

4) *The government introduces risk rating and creates adjustment interventions.* Under pressure from the managed care and financial services industries, its purpose is to act as a clearinghouse for health insurers and provider entities. The risk adjustments is very sophisticated, inexpensive genetic screening tests like a strategize MRSA screening, are available and are used in routinely in combination with traditional health risk appraisal methodologies to assess and individual's risk rating when he or she applied for health insurance.

5) *The consumer pays and chooses.* The individual consumer pays for trade-up in health plan choice, but the premium is paid for in variety of ways. large employers orchestrate health benefits for their employees on a defined-contribution basis.

6) *Providers focus on risk-*adjusted segments. Providers are paid a risk-adjusted monthly payment based on the pool of members signed on in any given month. Because providers have no incentive to cherry-pick recipients, they can focus on those types of patients they want to serve.

7) *E-commerce provides the infrastructures.* The health care system borrows much of the e-commerce infrastructure from financial services. A wide variety of e-health giants has emerged, including many financial service companies that migrate into health care, as well as health-care-specific e-commerce companies.

Green (1988) retorted that NHS public production and finance suggests that government should not attempt both to finance and produce health-care services. Instead, it should finance health care for those in need, to ensure that everyone has the power to buy health insurance cover, but it should not attempt to pay for all health-care services from taxation; it should regulate, refine, make and enforce the rules which enable a competitive market to serve interests of all, rich and poor alike; it should publish to enable people to make more effective choices.

In Green's book, he summarizes the NHS policy proposals in cognizant with tests screenings such as controlling Health Care Associated Infections e.g. MRSA:

- The NHS should be left intact, through pilot schemes to improve efficiency should be attempted.
- People dissatisfied with the NHS should be allowed to escape and to claim an age-weighted voucher representing the tax they had paid towards the NHS.
- They would required to relinquish their claim to free NHS services and to take out private insurance to the value of the voucher or more, including catastrophe cover.
- Privately insured individuals or families could receive care, including emergency treatment, from the NHS as paying customers and would not be confined to using private hospitals.
- Separate vouchers would be available for hospital care (excluding long stay) and primary care.
- The poor would receive a voucher sufficient to buy a specified set of health-care services.
- People opting out would take their voucher not direct to an insurance company but to a health purchase union, which would be responsible for making available several choices of insurance company.
- Most people would obtain cover through their employer or private association, but in addition statutory health purchase unions independent of government would established ultimately in each region.
- Insurance companies would be free to recruit individual subscribers, but they would not receive voucher payments unless the individual subscribed via a health purchase union.

There is another problem in NHS that the Health Act 2006 must addressed, this is the rationing of the waiting lists, according to Frankel and West (1993), the broadest view which emerges from the detailed examinations of waiting concerns the question of rationing finite health care resources. There is no question that rationing is inherent in the resourcing of health care provisions. Demand for health care may outstrip the resources made available such as health and social services, to be more specific the hospital facilities if these are available and accessible to the poor patients (under the bracket of low-income economic status), financial incentives and other medicinal benefits for poor patients, the numbers of doctors particular the specialist in certain health problems like heart surgeons et al (this could be exemplified by the ratio between doctors and patients on a national average) and so on and so forth. However, within this global pattern of scarcity, the finer analysis presented here suggests that long waiting times for some people and for some operations are not the consequence of any global mismatch between supply and demand but an expression of the implicit priorities within health care provision, which are themselves the product of range of organizational factors and professional preferences.

Frankel and West even expanded the discussion that rationing certainly exists in the National Health Services, as it does in any health care system. However the current system of rationing in Britain appears highly irrational in that the very conditions where comparatively cheap interventions are likely to lead to considerable health benefits are those selected for relative neglect. It is ironic that those very conditions, where a rational application of current resources could reasonably be expected to satisfy demand, are held up as evidence for the need for rationing.

The politics in NHS as Allsop (1995) argued created a 'command and control' model of health care that confabulated political interests. Government established the NHS as a result of democratic pressure and a Parliamentary mandate, the form was based on the provision of personal illness services within organizational hierarchy. Professional interest groups, particularly the medical profession, were involved in negotiations throughout and subsequently, the pattern of politics at national level was corporate. At the local level, the lack of central and managerial control allowed considerable professional autonomy. There are three questions in UK health care. The first is whether politics remains corporatist at the national level and whether there is discussion and agreement with the medical profession over policy developments. The second is whether the system of commissioning has reduced professional autonomy and social authority within the Trusts. The third is whether there are broader changes which will affect the cultural authority of medicine more generally. Answers to these questions can only be speculative as there is a dearth of empirical studies.

At the local level, where most doctors work, the politics of hospital work differs from that of general practice (GP), because within the GP, the health reforms have enhanced the power of political interests in relation to their hospital colleagues. In concluding remarks, the managed competition has introduced a new dynamic health care politics with insinuating the magnitude of MRSA infections and screening together with the medical mandate of NHS.

Hopefully primary and community care will continue to expand and the roles of the hospital reduce. This is likely to be accompanied by an increase in the range of specialist health care workers and the scope for self care by people themselves. A profound health care and social services must be established, wherein the local authorities may take over as purchasers of this welfare products in a democratic control unit in the health care system.

References:

Allsop, Judith (1995) *Foundations and Framework* (pp. 1-36) and *Health Policy in Britain: Towards the Twenty-first Century* (pp. 264-278) in *Health Policy and the NHS Towards 2000.* (2nd ed.) London: Longman.

Baines, Darrin L. and Whynes, David K. (1996) *Economics of Primary Care: Selection Bias in GP Fundholding.* (Vol. 5, No. 2 pp. 129-140) Health Economics: John Wiley & Sons, Ltd.

Beveridge, Sir William (1942) *Social Insurance and Allied Services.* (Presented to Parliament by Command of His Majesty) Referencing guide, http://www.sochealth.co.uk/history/beveridge.htm, Date accessed 2 December 2008.

Folland, Sherman, Goodman, Allen C., and Stano, Miron (2001) *The Relevance of Health Economics in Health Care* (pp. 1-19) in *The Economics of Health and Health Care.* New Jersey: Prentice-Hall, Inc.

Frankel, Stephen (Ed.) and West, Robert (1993) *What is to be Done?* (pp. 115-131) in *Rationing and Rationality in the National Health Service: The Persistence of Waiting Lists.* Basingstoke: Macmillan Press.

Gaucher, Ellen J., and Coffey, Richard J. (1993) *Reflections* (pp. 549-558) in *Total Quality in Health Care: From Theory to Practice.* San Francisco: Jossey-Bass Publishers.

Green, David G. (1988) *Getting from A to B* (pp. 71-89) in *Everyone a Private Patient: An Analysis of the Structural Flaws in the NHS and how they could be Remedied.* London: Institute of Economics Affairs.

Harrison, S., Hunter, D.J., and Pollitt, C. (1990) *The Dynamics of Health Policy* (pp. 153-163) in *The Dynamics of British Health Policy.* London: Routledge.

Harrison, Stephen et al. (1992) *Power and Culture in the National Health Service* (pp. 1-19) in *Just Managing: Power and Culture in the National Health Service.* Basingstoke: Macmillan Press.

Hawkes, Nigel (2007) *MRSA test on new patients reduces infections by 40%.* Referencing guide, http://www.timesonline.co.uk/tol/life_and_style/health/article3070736.ece, Date accessed 21 November 2008.

Kay A. (2002) *The Abolition of the GP Fundholding Scheme: A Lesson in Evidence-Based Policy Making.* (Vol. 52, No. 475, pp. 141-144) British Journal of General Practice: Royal College of General Practitioners.

Keshtgar M.R.S., Khalili A., and Coen PG, et al. (2007) *Impact of Rapid Molecular Screening for Meticillin-Resistant Staphylococcus aureus in Surgical Wards.* (pp. 381-386) London: John Wiley & Sons, Ltd.

Klevens, R. Monina (2007) *Invasive Meticillin-Resistant Staphylococcus aureus Infections in the United States.* (Vol. 298, No. 15, pp. 1763-1771) American Medical Assciation, CDC-Information Center.

McCaughey, Betsy (2006) *MRSA Screening Is Essential* (pp. 5-7) in *Unnecessary Deaths: The Human and Financial Costs of Hospital Infections.* (2nd ed.) New York: Committee to Reduce Infection Deaths, Inc.

Milio, Nancy (1991) *Making Healthy Public Policy: Developing the Science by Learning the Art: An Ecological Framework for Policy Studies* (pp. 7-28) in Badura, Bernhard and Kickbusch, Ilona (Ed.) *Promotion Health Research: Towards a New Social Epidemiology* (European Series, No. 37). England: WHO Regional Publications.

Morrison, Ian (2000) *Health Care in the New Millennium: The Long Boom Meets the Civil Society.* (pp. 213-230) in *Health Care in the New Millennium: Vision, Values, and Leadership.* San Francisco: Jossey-Bass Publishers.

National Health Service (2008) *Methicillin-resistant Staphylococcus aureus.* Referencing guide, http://www.nhs.uk/conditions/mrsa/Pages/Introduction.aspx?url=Pages/What-is-it.aspx, Date accessed 21 November 2008.

Nicholson, D., McLoughlin, L., and Mills, H. (2007) *Methicillin Resistant Staphylococcus Aureus (MRSA) for Community Settings.* (pp. 1-16) Referencing guide, http://Bristol\Website\InfectionControl\MRSAOct07.doc, Date accessed 21 November 2008., Bristol Primary Care Trust (National Health Service).

MRSA Action UK (2008) *Mission Statement on Methicillin-Resistant Staphylococcus aureus.* Referencing guide, http://www.mrsaactionuk.net/, Date accessed 21 November 2008.

Rao, Gopal (2008) *Prevalence and Risk Factors for Methicillin-resistant Staphylococcus aureus in adult emergency admissions: A case for Screening all Patients.* Referencing guide, http://www.sciencedirect.com, Date accessed 21 November 2008.

Siegel, Jane D. et al (2006) *Management of Multidrug-Resistant Organisms in Healthcare Settings.* (pp. 1-33) Department of Health & Human Services, USA.

Stevens, Janice (2008) *Reducing MRSA and other Healthcare Associated Infections.* Referencing guide, http://www.clean-safe-care.nhs.uk, Date accessed 21 November 2008.

Verar, Wilfredo Jr., M. (2008) *Comparison of Selected Phenotypic Assays and MecA-PCR in Detecting Methicillin Resistance in Clinical Isolates of Staphylococcus aureus.* (Thesis, Abstract) Quezon City: University of the Philippines-Diliman Press.

Wikipedia's page (2008) *Methicillin-resistant Staphylococcus aureus.* Referencing guide, http://en.wikipedia.org/wiki/Methicillin-resistant_Staphylococcus_aureus, Date accessed 21 November 2008.